Prof. Arnold Ehret's

THUS SPEAKETH THE STOMACH
AND
THE TRAGEDY OF NUTRITION

Introduced & Edited by Prof. Spira

PROF. ARNOLD EHRET'S
THUS SPEAKETH THE STOMACH
AND
THE TRAGEDY OF NUTRITION

By Prof. Arnold Ehret (1866-1922)

Introduced and Edited by Prof. Spira

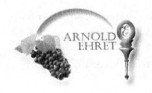

Copyright Breathair Publishing

Columbus, Ohio

2nd Edition 2014

Email: info@mucusfreelife.com

General Disclaimer: The content found in this document and related websites is based upon the opinions and research of the authors and is strictly for informational and educational purposes only. If you choose to use the material in this book on yourself, the authors and publishers take no responsibility for your actions and decisions or the consequences thereof. The content is not intended to replace a one-on-one relationship with a qualified health care professional and is not intended as medical advice. It is intended as a sharing of knowledge, information about health, and opinions based on the research and experiences of the authors and their collaborators.

Breathair Publishing
Columbus, Ohio
Printed by CreateSpace, an Amazon.com Company
CreateSpace, Charleston SC

Available from www.mucusfreelife.com, Amazon.com, Kindle, and other retail outlets

Printed in the United States of America

Second Edition, 2014

ISBN-13: 978-0-99-065644-9
ISBN-10: 0-99-065644-6

www.mucusfreelife.com

Discover other titles by Breathair Publishing

Spira Speaks: Dialogs and Essays on the Mucusless Diet Healing System

Prof. Arnold Ehret's Rational Fasting for Physical, Mental and Spiritual Rejuvenation: Introduced and Edited by Prof. Spira

The Definite Cure of Chronic Constipation and Overcoming Constipation Naturally: Introduction by Prof. Spira

Coming Soon

Art of Transition: Spira's Mucusless Diet Healing System Menu and Recipe Guide

CONTENTS

Introduction

Professor Arnold Ehret was a German healer, dietitian, philosopher, teacher, visionary, and one of the first people to advocate fasting and a plant-based, vegan, mucus-free lifestyle as a therapy for healing. For over 100 years, his written works and teachings have touched the lives of thousands of health seekers pursuing higher levels of vitality. He was also a cultural icon who had a great influence on the "Back-to-Nature" counter-cultural movement which first emerged in Victorian Era Europe, and then migrated to Southern California in the early 1900s. The movement fundamentally influenced the hippie counter-culture of the 1960s.

In the early 1900s, Ehret opened a hugely popular sanitarium in Ascona, Switzerland where he treated and cured thousands of patients considered incurable by the so-called "medical authorities." During the latter part of the decade, Ehret engaged in a series of fasts monitored by German and Swiss officials. Within a period of 14 months, Ehret completed a fast of 21 days, one of 24 days, one of 32 days, and one of 49 days. He became one of the most in-demand health lecturers, journalists, and educators in Europe as he saved the lives of thousands of people.

On June 27, 1914, just before World War I, Ehret left from Bremen for the United States to see the Panama Exposition and sample the fruits of the continent. He found his way to California, which was viewed as an "Eden of the West." The region was also

1

undergoing a horticultural renaissance due to botanists like Luther Burbank, which greatly interested Ehret. The war prevented him from returning to Germany and he settled in Mount Washington where he prepared his manuscripts and diplomas in his cultivated eating gardens. With the help of Fred Hirsch, he founded Ehret Literature and began to publish his masterful works.

Today, Ehret's works are increasing in popularity as people learn of the healing power of plant-based, vegan, and raw-food diets. Overall, Ehret believes that pus- and mucus-forming foods are unnatural for humans to eat. He asserts that a diet of fruits and green, leafy vegetables, i.e., mucus-free foods, are the most healing and powerful foods for humans. The world needs Ehret's work now more than ever. In an era where people consume genetically modified, mucus-forming *frankenfoods* daily, the simplicity and truthfulness of Ehret's teachings can transform humanity for the better.

If your intestines could talk, what would they say? What if you could understand health through the perspective of your stomach? In this unprecedented work, Arnold Ehret first gives voice to the stomach and then reveals the foundation of human illness. In this version, minor edits have been made to correct existing errors and outdated gendered syntax.

—*Prof. Spira (2013)*

Forward

We read in the Bible, Genesis 1:29: "I have given you every herb bearing seed which is upon the earth—and every tree in which is the fruit yielding seed; to you it shall be for meat." You will note that the word "meat" is used to denote human's "food"; not the carcass of dead animals! Arnold Ehret was a student and follower of Nature's laws—in communion with GOD! The Ehret teachings have their foundation in TRUTH—but until they are "demonstrated," the average individual cannot grasp their significance and consequently—not until then—do they prove acceptable to the great majority!

Arnold Ehret described and denounced superstition and ignorance; but like similar teachings of great men, his teachings have been grossly misunderstood by the average individual and unjustly criticized by many health teachers. It has now been well over 70 years that his voice was first heard vainly sounding a note of warning, desperately hoping to dispel the colossal ignorance of the average uninformed individual concerning Natural laws! His teachings have opened many new avenues of healing, and his wonderful philosophy and knowledge offered to those willing to accept bring thousands of new converts each year, from every part of the globe!

Ehret taught that the mind governs all organic action of the physical body instinctively, and we therefore find humankind gradually evolving from the primitive stage to a higher intellectual plane. The physical and mental welfare of millions of individuals living today are desperately searching for a truthful presentation of this knowledge found only in Prof. Arnold Ehret's message and it is therefore eagerly awaited by an expectant world! Is it asking too much that you lay aside preconceived ideas, opinions, or prejudices and read the Ehret articles with an open mind, particularly his article "Tragedy of Nutrition." Hopefully the truth will eventually dawn upon you, possibly months after reading—for some portion may have indelibly stamped an imprint on your mind—and intuitively proven its correctness!

There is no "mystery" connected with Ehret's "Mucusless Diet" theory—though it differs almost entirely from other "healing systems," especially his lucid explanations. Ehret practiced no deception; his statements are easily understood because of their outstanding "simplicity" of expression. He continually informs the student, "whatsoever is not simple—easily understood—is 'false' and therefore not the truth!"

Fundamentally, Ehret's teachings of his philosophy are basically the love of NATURE itself—love of all outdoors! The love of flowers and trees, the love of all of the birds and animals! Ehret loved the sunshine and the rain, the cold and the warmth, the bright days and the cloudy days. And he sincerely taught that we must feel justly proud of our own physical bodies, CLEAN both internally and externally!

Our "love" of birds and four-legged animals instinctively warns that we must not harm these fellow creatures—and never kill them for our food! Mother Nature has abundantly supplied us with quantities of delicious, nutritious fruits and vegetables on which we thrive! With a clean bloodstream coursing through our bodies, any thought of cannibalism becomes obnoxious.

Arnold Ehret taught tolerance! Respect for the rights of others and acceptance of their rights to their own beliefs! Never attempt to force others to accept your beliefs, but rather through precept and example create a desire on the part of those interested in health to seek this great truth of their own free will! Through your tolerance of

4

"ignorance" you will have proven your superiority, and eventually'
"nonbelievers" will see the bright glow of TRUTH!

—Fred S. Hirsch, DNS. (*Ehret Literature*)

Thus Speaketh the Stomach
By Prof. Arnold Ehret

The philosopher Immanuel Kant and other contemporary thinkers have ventured to critically investigate the process of thinking itself. The more modern, materialistic school may at least claim the merit of having reminded us that normal thinking requires a normal organ of thought, with well-organized brain convolutions. Materialism placed the carriers of philosophical minds upon earthly soil again. It did not commence its speculations in the background, nor in the abstract, super-sensual, and metaphysical—it put the scalpel of its thinking, figuratively and in reality at the organs of the soul, and opened up a philosophy of life—starting with the material atom, and the cell of living substances. Brain convolutions, and the quality of nerve substance, seemed to become the criterion of a material basis—in order to obtain a "Critique of Pure Reason," without sophistic tendencies, and to grasp the spiritual and physical life—the process of thinking, as perception, logic, and judgment. Now, the cell appeared really tangible and visible, as a specifically organized unit of living substance and as a coordinated carrier of bodily and mental functions. The anatomy of these microorganisms is known; but the quality of their functions, the causes of their vitality, are yet obscure. They forget that all depends upon the nourishing with live blood, and that the fundamental lever of all thinking—of thinking, itself—has to be put at the stomach, the center of blood formation—if we want to solve the mystery of life. One has to go to the gravity center of the organism—that is, one's stomach—in order to understand, alleviate, remedy the heaviness, the impediments to one's functions, known as disease. One has to look into the workings and at the basis of their central organs if they want to find the cause of accelerated and lowered functional capacity of all parts of the whole system, which are being nourished with blood, by the stomach.

Jean-Jacques Rousseau dictated his writings while in a recumbent position. Freidrich Von Schiller put his feet into cold water while writing. Fainting is often the last stage of a bloodless condition of the brain, caused through a full stomach. Pythagoras had to fast 40 days in order to understand the wisdom of Egypt. However, not because fasting causes a bloodless condition of the brain, as is generally believed, but because the very opposite is the case. Far better than recumbent—as with Rousseau—or by cooling the feet—as with Schiller—does the human brain produce the best thoughts, the surest perceptions, when thoroughly permeated with blood. If, by fasting—as with Pythagoras—the stomach has been brought to that state of cleanliness whereby perfect digestion of food is assured, there will be no interference in the regular nourishing of the brain with blood through the presence of auto-toxins. One has eventually to begin at the stomach with a blood purifying. We must enter upon a higher grade of health starting from the center of blood formation in order to obtain a perception of "blood-pure reason" a priori that disease in the main is but an unconscious laying of mines in the body, which will be brought to an inflammation and eruption through secondary, incident causes such as a cold, infection, etc. We must eliminate the presence of unevacuated feces, retained through sticky mucus in the pockets of the intestines, constantly poisoning, and thereby interfering with proper digestion and blood building.

Not only all life, but all culture in the better sense, proceeds from the stomach. But this organ, through false nursing by the too-material cult of Bacchus and Lucullus—according to Nietsche—has become the father of all misery; the secret hotbed of all disease. Here a latent deposit of moribund matter, consisting of retained waste products, is acting oppressively on the brain and corrupting the blood, and in each special case of disease, besides being the direct cause coming from the obscure, underground stomach cover, it obscures the clinical picture of every symptom of an eliminative nature, for the time being. As can be proved, pounds of the secret, pathological ailment are deposited within the tissues as a primary cause of disease; as chronic corruption of the blood—coming from the underground, the obscure unknown, the mysterious X—in the course of all acute and chronic disease processes.

If today in some manner I may introduce a speaking stomach, this is done for three reasons: First, because this rather antiquated form of expression seems better adapted to impart personal perceptions and concepts. Second, because the functions of an organ—a process of Nature! a force; a will; the sense and purposeful intentions of unconscious partial functions of the human body—when especially personified and given speech, are brought nearer to the general intelligence of the people. Third, because diet and with that the stomach—the blood formation—are the first things implied in the question: "What and how should we eat and drink in order to get well and remain healthy?" Perhaps even science can find some animating thoughts in this idea.

Supported by an extensive material of facts and by certain experiments upon my own body—such as no one else has made, so far—I will attempt to introduce to you the stomach—as the gathering place of that pathological material that has generally been called encumbrance, auto-toxins, morbid disposition, or tendency, without the presence of which the action of a secondary cause of disease is impossible. I have made experiments to produce a cold, to get malaria infection, etc., with a negative result; but quickly eliminated it after a thorough removal of the first general cause—consisting of the complete encumbrance—through the stomach by fasting and using my own diet. In order to put disease, as an experiment, upon a common basis, I went to the limit of endangering my life. In a state of improved health, I would intentionally eat myself sick, to a certain extent, in order to eat myself surely and radically well again—for my own satisfaction. To my knowledge, this has

9

never before been attempted. If science does not care about this experimenting of mine—it may continue to look on, smilingly, at what is to follow. I, myself, believe I shall thereby be of service to the sick—to the life efficiency of the human race—to the promotion of the people's vigor, and to all humanity.

And now, let the stomach speak in the principal role of the "Tragedy of Human Nutrition."

Thus Speaketh the Stomach:

"Histogenetically, I am, at first, a primitive, intestinal cell; a tiny, hollow bag with a mouth-opening; this being the ultimate, common, basic form of all true multi-cellular vertebrates, according to Haeckel. In the whole scale of living animal organisms up to and including humans, I am located in the center, at the point of gravity. To me— the Stomach—belongs this centrally located place; for I am the single building spot; the organized working apparatus for raw material, and at the same time, the master builder. I get my orders through the brain—the chief management—as unconscious instincts from the world's architect. To me, alone—with my assistant, the bloodstream—belongs, in the main, the material building of the whole body; the formation and shaping of the organs, their maintenance, and the supply of repair material. I am the material main center of growth, replenishing and working the whole organism. Even the chief management—the brain—is subject to my food carrier, the blood. I have always been and shall remain the first and absolute ruler in the cell state of humans and of animals. To me belongs the center of being and health; of pain and disease, and of passing away. Thus I, only, in the first line, can be the source and supply of remedy—the hotbed and the deathbed of disease.

"In the chase after causative factors of disease, I have been displaced from my dominating position among the organs, in human's perception—however, in the scale of so-called pleasures of life and culture; I have been elevated to the 'Chief God.' In reality, the millenarian mistreatment of humans has made of me a dark chamber of suicidal table enjoyment—and pain, my warning voice and defensive force, has been choked in the endless courses of

10

dimmed kitchens. Human's thinking has become obscured in the tempo of overculture of their abdomen—the conception of health has dissolved in fancy—and the specter of disease is haunting him. Also the terror of this phantom, their suffering and death, emanate from me. If I am the center of life; why should I not also be the center of death?

"Pain, uneasiness in general—and in particular parts—are my signals to 'Stop too much unnecessary eating!' These are alarm dispatches, and indicate functional disturbances in the vascular system, as a reaction on me,—which I ingeniously support by loss of appetite. They answer me by strangling my voice through more eating. My voice works as a danger signal, causing pain—because, through overeating and drinking, the pressure and density of blood are increased by me, instead of being diminished. In the state of disease and elimination, the bloodstream carries the dissolved auto-toxins from me to the kidneys; this goes on painlessly, with relaxed tissues only while fasting—which acts as a relief. Pain is merely my cry of distress; an expression of my disturbed healing work, which I can perform thoroughly only when I am empty and fasting. In fact and truth, my pain signals are good and life promoting, thought and action provoking to thinking people. They should be the refining fire, the upward move for the overcoming of suffering and disease—the forerunner of a new dawn of life. (These ideas may serve as a contribution to the Philosophy of Suffering; or Revelation of all values.)

"I, the Stomach, am the primary ruler over life and death, from the first primitive intestinal cell to the passing away of the last creature. My rule over living beings is self-evident—as I am the first deciding court of remedy, of repair, of restoration of the functional and organic disturbances called disease. Unceasingly, with the help of the organs of elimination and protection, I am secretly at work to regulate the well-being of humans with Edenic reserve forces. Especially in advanced years, I maintain a secret process of life-protecting and life-sustaining purpose in the most subtle form. Under continued inflow of inassimilable matter, of so-called food culture, and especially during the stoppage of my drainage canal, I am unable

11

to maintain the balance. I become flabby from the eliminating work, and so does the whole tissue and blood system of my surroundings and of the entire body. I can neither digest the inflow, nor overcome it by secretion. I have to deposit matter for more tranquil times, and store it up in the tissues. Abnormal distension of my cavity and of the whole body is called 'vigorous health,'—which must be registered by a pathological condition.

"My 'striking' and the possibility of eliminating the morbid matter of putrescent refuse consists in absolute emptiness and sobriety of fasting—and on an instinctive animal command, of the 'world regisseur.' My intention is good—a regulating of the health and running activity—a sort of self-defense,—an aid from the underground. Instead of properly defending yourselves against all enemies and dangers of life, you have throttled my life and healing activities, my digestive power, and my eating capacity. My glands, my walls, the tissues of my surroundings, and especially my 10-meter-long canal are permeated, infected, soiled in proportion to my chronic abuse, through modern eating. At the basis of my tissues, especially those of my surroundings, I have to deposit the residue, which in the course of all disease remains unknown to you as the primary cause—because only while I am empty and fasting can I attack it, devour it, work it off, burn it up, and healingly eliminate it through the bloodstream.

"Instead of being a fountain of wholesome life—the source of purest blood and health—I have become the secret underground chamber, the breeding place of all suffering, and the father of all misery.

"Thus I take up my 'song of lamentation,' as the most temperate representative of the present time." He that hath ears to hear, let him hear.' Already, in the womb of the mother—out of care for a new human life—I induce disgust for unnatural 'cultured' eating—to retain the purity of the blood, and to conform to the instinct for primitive nutrition through fruit. However, I am fed double rations— and they wonder why the birth takes place with pain and danger to life for mother and child. I am given food poor in minerals, especially in lime—such as flesh, boiled, decalcified milk—while I long for the lime salts of fruits—since I have to build up a new bony frame for the embryo. I catch up every milligram of lime salts, even at the expense of the mother's teeth, in order to give it to the child in formation. Hysteria and caries of the teeth of the pregnant is how they diagnose my care for a new human life. I am unable to build good mother's milk substance since I am lacking in fruit sugar, its main ingredient—although I am flooded with cow's milk. I am also kept well supplied with this during the nursing period of the young one—also with the entire list of imaginable slime preparations. I cannot overcome the cheesy, putrescent refuse, and the slimy condition reaches from the throat to the pasted and clogged-up outlet. My interior is stuffed with boiled, pallid, curdled, and decalcified milk, and its germ-producing condition threatens to strangle the windpipe of the little one. I am laboring with obstructions, impediments, and friction in fever heat. By forceful, downward pressure I try to make room, but my good intentions are frustrated through constipating drugs. Now I have the emergency vents of the skin open to throw off waste and impurities that slide into the bloodstream.

"Measles, scarlet fever, eruptions—they call my last efforts to throw off the morbid, the useless, the disease germs. If, in spite of all, the young citizen succeeds in getting on his legs, he at once searches for sweets and fruits, to which I urge him, with Edenic instinct. The live elements of fruit sugar give me a chance for a radical discharge of the putrescent mucus masses that have accumulated into a dangerous breeding field within myself—with a stench reminding one of carrion and death. I discharge the first layer of my own depository of disease, and that of the intestines, as a warning to reform and as a sign of my good intentions as to 'life insurance.' This is called loose stool, scientifically known as diarrhea and colitis, and is stopped by opium. Since my evacuations originate from putrid, curdled milk, they are of greenish color. With adults, especially with heavy meat eaters, they are blackish. In extreme cases of my defense work, downward as well as upward, they speak more learnedly of Cholera morbus. If through climatic heat the danger of

13

fermentation is still greater, and my provisional eruptions more intense, then my attempts at cleansing from slime and bacillus soil is called Cholera Asiatica—with which one usually smothers in their own morass because he counteracts my eliminative efforts. When attempting to gradually accustom my youthful purity to meat, liquors, etc., I respond, in the child, with squeamishness, and, in my juvenile elasticity, I try to eject the loathsome, unnatural stuff, through energetic contractions. This is called 'colic,' and with the aid of the rod, they force the reactive youngster to weaken my original power, through so-called strengthening food.

"At the age of puberty, I start my special effort at cleansing, with the woman—in the organ of gestation—to take place regularly each month, before the period of possible conception, with the sole purpose of cleansing before fecundation. This phenomenon is the health-regulating process of disease and is lessened both as to quantity and frequency in proportion to the general efforts at cleansing; commencing with me. It becomes superfluous and disappears entirely with perfect health—if I am fed exclusively on pure and unmixed food, with fruit alone. (For proof, we refer to the lives of many saints.) I am likewise interested in the formation of pure blood in the young man, since the quality of his blood is not only of importance to him, but to his whole future generation. The sins of the ancestors and the germs of immortality are in the atmosphere of today, but, with me, nobody has dared to find them. The entire list of sexuo-pathological symptoms may be pretty closely produced through a one-sided, extreme increase in feeding on 'food of the beasts of prey.' Do you know that you can kill a person by feeding them exclusively on flesh—the much-lauded main food of the century?

"With the Stomach, also, 'talking amounts to silver,' while silence is often worth gold, especially when one's stomach could speak whole volumes about the foolishness of people, but without avail. To the asthmatic I give timely warnings of my uneasiness due to lack of oxygen in the digestion. I control the elimination and subsequent emaciation in these types, especially. "Tuberculosis has a certain healing tendency," said Prof. Virchow, the great pathologist. This

14

disease also originates with me—in the underground—destroying the air organ when I cannot get any more air on account of wrong eating. To overcome the highest degree of blood corruption and the breakdown of the entire cell state—as in the case of tuberculosis and cancer—my bloodstream seeks to get a crater-like eruption spot and an emergency vent, as it were, to throw off the products of decay, viz, slime and pus. At the very beginning, before the process of eruption, I ulcerate the surroundings while depositing, germinating, and rebuilding—for the filth is of especially putrefactive origin— resulting from excessive consumption of flesh and eggs. In most cases of this kind, I—the builder of the body of humans—am unable to be of material help—and if they attempt to assist me with their 'best diet,' they only make things worse.

"Do they not even try to regulate the heartbeat through means which I have to take? Then why should not I also be the 'father of tortured hearts,' when I, through high pressure, must poison and current the blood which is banked up in the chambers of this valve, congesting the air pump (the lungs) where gas—oxygen—is lacking? Not only must I, as the breeding and blood-forming place produce germs of putrefaction in the field of underground encumbrance, but by force of emergency, the pathological matter even forms into crystallized, stony condensations obstructing the bloodstream in narrow passageways (as in the case of rheumatism) or being deposited as stones in the gall bladder, or in the notches of the intestines.

"The resisting bulwark and greatest counterforce, the greatest impediment that makes it possible to prevent this germ depositary of all diseases is chronic constipation, the obstruction of the end of my drainage pipe—the rectum. Of the upper portion of my auxiliary organ—the intestinal canal—only one part need be mentioned here. In sheer blindness, they mistook the appendix for a 'blind,' superfluous, and even impending structure, which, however, was to assist in the lubrication and smoothening of the chyle through its secretion—like the oiler of a machine. Naturally, a machine will run for a time with a clogged-up oiler or without same—but only until it becomes burning hot.

15

"Still greater than within myself and my surroundings is the accumulation of filth at the outlet of the drainage pipe. Through decades of damming up, there has gathered a mire-like mass beyond description. The deep folds conceal heaps of slime and fecal matter in stony formation of many years' standing. This ulcerating and fermenting depositary of putrefying refuse of the process of disintegration of one's own tissues is, in conjunction with myself, a first-class hotbed and breeding place of all diseases. Here is the dark, secret, underground reservoir of the dietary mire, which is poisoning the bloodstream from childhood on, and like an obscure subterranean spring, is feeding all painful disease symptoms. There we find the deeper causes of apoplexy, neurasthenia, typhus, head troubles, kidney and liver affections,—and of the varied list of 'specialties' invented by the 'medical brain.' I, the principal organ of digestion, like all other parts, especially the injured tissues of blood vessels congested by a cold, continuously receive from this reservoir deadly excremental gases and substances through the circulation— and I even stir up this partially dead chamber within a living body because I must, naturally, expel my contents there into.

"Germs of decayed and live parasites, broods of vermin of various species, live and thrive on the refuse of flesh and starch in the alimentary canals of unnumbered people displaying a good appetite and a voracity for the favored food of these pests. Fruit acids would kill them—but my interior walls and my reflecting image, the taste-organ (tongue), are so charged with slime and so pasty that I cannot make known my primitive instinct for fruit. Air, water, sunshine, fruit sugar, fruit acids,—and the building stones of organized substances containing albumen in the maximum of one-half per cent, were originally and still are the sole and natural components of my helio-electric formation of blood—with radioactive force from sweet scents and odors of fruits, 'the bread of Heaven.'

"I was originally tuned to a mono-diet consisting of a varied selection from the fruits in season, differing in the degree of their water value and in accordance with the position of the sun and the average temperature of the respective zones. Out of these, I produced force and warmth, bone and muscle, for Edenic humans,

16

healthy and free from disease germs—just as today with the frugivorous apes or with quadrupeds, on grass and water, in twenty degrees below zero.

"I can ward off and expel the much-accused poisons of modern civilization, such as alcohol, coffee, tobacco, etc., in much less time than I can throw off the ballast of 'cultured' eating, which has become the custom. The continuous overloading therewith, in disgusting mixtures and without necessity, threatens to choke and drown me and my life functions. Within me, on a base of soups, beer, and wine, there is constantly swimming a varied and heterogeneous mixture of unchewed and useless substances, which are already largely decomposed—out of which I am supposed to turn out the live ingredients of the blood.

"The first thing to do would be to value all eatables accordingly so that none of the necessary secretions and excretions would adhere to me or to any part of the digestive apparatus, encumbering and obstructing everything with pasty slime—and to liberate me, first of all, from all slime permeating my structure—through the use of dissolving foods, especially fruits, salads and vegetables.

"To be or not to be healthy or sick—the life and death of humans and humanity lies within my power. I am the ultimate smithery and destiny to all humans. According to natural law and purpose, I am the hammer that can fashion out of blood and iron men with vigorous, indestructible health. To be sure, it takes live blood made out of the meat of grapes, oranges, and such fruits full of organic iron—instead of dead animals, with disintegrated and devitalized albuminous matter. I seem only to have become the anvil on which they think to weld dead matter into live substance. My silent, Edenic harmony has been turned into dull growling. I already spit sparks of fire, which will consume him who means to throttle me. Their downfall is my paternal blood on the stage of life, in the *Tragedy of Human Nutrition*.

"Thus sounds my lamentation: I and my auxiliary organs have been proven, in the zoological order of evolution—with 'moral glory'—to be the organs of beasts of prey—and, in the biological

17

order, from a dietetic and physiological standpoint, we have been out on a level with the swine—in order to justify the modern diet. All species and varieties I must digest, from the mollusks of the sea to the ruminants of the field and the birds of the air—and I have, apparently, adapted myself to their form of nutrition. Humans have lost the appetite for fruits—the primary diet of the human stomach—and the faith in their live power (according to Mr. Birher-Benner.) The genealogy of humankind may be traced back to the ape family, through a queer branching off—but, in the present condition of my auxiliary organs, the teeth, and intestines, and of myself, my brotherly similarity to the frugivorous ape, in regard to diet, has been denied.

"Humans were formerly content to be satisfied with a few fruits of the forest, in order to procreate god-like, Edenic human beings, as the predecessors of the hunter, with spear and fire. I still exist on this prehistoric reserve fund of force, while dissipating my capital fund in the digestion of luxuries. My present silence—while being fed on milk, eggs, flesh, cereals and pulses, liquors, and the entire modern artificial diet, speaks volumes. My glands and the introductory structures of my tract are clogged with a slimy, sticky mucus, which has ruined them. The sensory and defensory nerves are benumbed. With the patience of a giant, I endure the ten-fold measure and carrion-like quality of the meals, lauded as good and strengthening—while they are the very opposite, weakening and inducing incapacity to react against inassimilable matter. In fact, I operate under great difficulties and 'keep the machine going' with the most necessary water and air. They call my silence under the strain of desperate effort—and the mute patience of a giant—'good digestion.' While the organic wheel is jarring, heaving, and groaning, and the pipes threaten to burst.

"Grapes, cherries, apples, all sweet and sour fruits I easily digest and turn into pure blood through my Edenic capacities—only when I have thereby eliminated and ejected the last remnant of refuse matter accumulated during a lifetime. If you again extend the hand of reconciliation for the 'bread of Heaven' and you want to eat yourself well, then I commence the most ingenious mining work with the new blood from the sun kitchen. With it, I work through the whole body, stirring up the old, latent disease germs, and especially the new-symptom fields. I begin the healing and transmutation of the entire human. The most radical cleansing of myself and of my surroundings—particularly of my drainage system, which is full of retained refuse matter, furnishing the real reduction of the entire encumbrance—and manifesting itself in an alarming emaciation. However, I can only commence my constructive, nourishing work with fruits, after all worn-out building material of my mansion has been removed. I can then, only, become again the fountain of health, the wall of life, the inexhaustible source of vigor and pleasure—although hereditarily since Adam, through millenniums, and, individually, for decades, I have been the father of misery and the germinating center of all diseases and afflictions."

"THUS SPEAKETH THE STOMACH."

- FINIS -

THE TRAGEDY OF NUTRITION
By Prof. Arnold Ehret

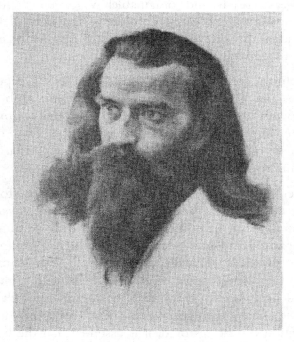

Sketch from original photograph of

Arnold Ehret taken at the end of a 40-day fast

Life Is a Tragedy of Nutrition

Nature's voice inspires those willing to listen to her teachings to a spiritual veneration and deep respect for our Creator! The power of health, beauty, grace, truth, and wisdom, everlastingly immune to all forms of disease, is probably one of the most sought after attainments of humans. But the habit of eating, striking all civilized humankind, involves and proves the saying I coined many years ago—"Life is a Tragedy of Nutrition." Humans of today must constantly eat merely to assuage the pains caused through elimination of poisons accumulated in the stomach!

And to those willing to listen and give heed to the undeniable voice of Mother Nature, it becomes simple, for all of these blessings are within easy reach and obtainable! Vigorous health, lifelong usefulness, and a happy, carefree future is the rightful heritage of every individual promising a happier and spiritually enlightened future, with that greatly desired longevity a certainty.

My teachings are "old" yet "NEW"; hopefully acceptable to all truth seekers anxious to participate in the supreme embodiment of abundant, joyous health! The fundamental truth that we must all first learn is the importance of obedience to the laws of Nature. Humankind of today seems indifferent to the great harm done to both body and soul through eating unnatural foods.

Health culture has always been a matter of religion, for the body and soul are difficult to separate. We find priests and physicians were generally one and the same person! But the truly Natural mode of living was ignored and now practically forgotten. Primitive humans were strong physically, mentally, and spiritually. For many centuries past, behind the walls of secluded cloisters, meal eating, gluttony, and drunkenness held full sway. Many false doctrines which originated through these unnatural environments are still accepted today! Before proper nutrition can be restored, it is essential that the bloodstream be improved and regenerated, in order that it might, after dissolving and eliminating the disease deposits contained in every tissue of the body, successfully carry away these poisons and waste.

22

When I first became interested in dietetics and followed a strict vegetarian life, my food intake consisted mainly of starchy vegetables, wheat products, "nourishing" nut preparations, and all of the dairy products, i.e., milk, butter, cheese, and eggs. In fact, drinking milk regularly with each meal was scrupulously carried out, only to find that my physical condition became worse and worse!

Stimulants in daily use, such as alcohol, coffee, tea, cocoa, tobacco, and spices, together with sugar and salt, are "poisons," so we are told, and should be avoided! My present attitude toward these so-called "poisons" has changed considerably. Stimulants and condiments, if continually used, will undoubtedly affect the nervous system. BUT, they most certainly are not solid obstructions, nor do they leave sticky wastes or mucus stored up in the human body, which occurs when unnatural and wrong foods such as starchy foods and dairy products, i.e., milk, butter, cheese, and eggs are eaten, all of which play such an important part in the vegetarian diet. I have found that condiments are far less harmful than gluttony, so that compared to overeating they are practically harmless. They stimulate more or less, at the expense of vitality and the efficiency of the nerves, but as stated above, they do not produce, nor do they leave, any substantial amount of waste in the body as do all of the wheat products, starch foods, and the meat, fats, and dairy products.

Admittedly, alcohol is surely a "poison," but the English physician, Dr. S. Graham, originator of Graham flour, certainly struck the nail squarely on the head when he wrote, "A drunkard may become old. But a glutton NEVER!" Every centenarian that I have ever known used alcohol moderately—and a few were even heavy users of tobacco. But without exception, all of the centenarians were very, very restrictive eaters—in fact, the total amount of their daily food intake would scarcely keep a bird alive! And here we uncover and reveal the evident secret of longevity—RESTRICT YOUR FOOD INTAKE TO A MINIMUM! Many of the saints of the Catholic Church lived to a ripe old age, and records show that they lived on only a "handful of food" a day!

23

So much is sure—there are not two known truths regarding the physical and spiritual perfectness of the human being. I have shown by "classic" examples that the highest degree of real civilization of mental and spiritual standards was attained and could be reached only through a most perfect body, enjoying splendid, superb health in every line: the result of physical culture, dietetics, and fasting. No individual can hope to attain this much desired state if they fail to free their minds of all superstition, nor properly care for their bodies in accordance with Nature's methods in every respect. They cannot hope to be saved from disease and imperfectness. Humankind all over the world must soon take up—in the broadest way—a program of care of the body and physical culture, patterned exactly like that followed in the classic age of ancient Greece, and from that alone will depend the salvation of our present civilization!

A "sudden" or "too rapid" change from the "wrong" foods to an exclusive fruit diet often causes undesirable disturbances, even in the body of an entirely healthy individual. It is therefore preferable that the change from today's accepted diet of meat, bread, and potatoes be accomplished through following the Transition Diet as taught in my book, the *Mucusless Diet Healing System*. While it is true that you may experience a more "vigorous" feeling during the first few days of an exclusive fruit diet, it often happens that a feeling of weakness, fatigue accompanied by headaches, and even heart palpitation set in. This is caused through the loosening and dissolving of "poisons," filth, and morass that the body has accumulated over the years through "overeating" and that are now being eliminated through the circulating bloodstream. This can easily cause more or less systemic disturbances, and unless you are thoroughly convinced of the efficacy of a natural diet, you can easily become dissuaded to a point where you will not only question, but actually lose all faith, in continuing with further attempts to accomplish this necessary internal purification. It is for this reason that the "healing crises" must be understandably recognized and carried on. The appearance of a "haggard face" or a feeling of "general depression" must not cause you to lose sight of the ultimate goal you are anxious to achieve—the hoped-for GOOD HEALTH!

Thousands of seriously ill persons have succeeded in overcoming their ailments through following a "non-breakfast" plan alone! Two meals a day has proven ample for the average individual. The "breakfast" or first meal can be eaten at 10:00 a.m. and the next meal as early as 4:30 p.m. or whatever later time proves more convenient. There are also many followers of the one-meal-a-day plan—and they prefer their meal in the late afternoon. They at least receive the benefit of a 24-hour fast, since no solid food of any kind is eaten between meals. Liquids (water, fruit, and vegetable juices) can be used anytime, if or when desired.

My mucusless diet consists of starchless vegetables and fruits. With this knowledge, you can choose and combine food correctly— and the possession of another important truth of life is now revealed to you!

Meat-eating animals, being carnivorous by nature, require freshly killed meat for their daily subsistence, which explains why the "domesticated" animals fed exclusively on cooked meats without the fresh blood and bones eventually become ill and die. Laboratory tests feeding a diet of "refined" white flour to rats and mice soon cause these animals to die!

During my stay in Egypt and Turkey, I cannot recall having met a "nervous person," yet almost without exception the inhabitants of these countries smoked almost continuously and drank strong coffee at the same time! The secret seemed obvious—they were as whole very light eaters. And practically no meat at all was eaten by them. Careful observations of myself and many of my patients convinced me that foods such as meat, starches, and dairy products are more directly to blame for nerve disturbances and so-called "heart trouble," rather than the use of coffee, tea, chocolate, and tobacco. Please do not misunderstand these statements and assume that I am defending these products, for they most assuredly should be classified as "poisons!" I am merely trying to show that the "nerve poisons" could have resulted through other sources. When the individual suffering from a nervous breakdown attempts to go on an exclusive sweet or acid-type fruit diet, the effect upon them will be the same as would result from drinking tea or coffee, proving conclusively that wastes and poisons in the systems are the direct cause of their "nervous breakdown." My teachings clearly prove that knowledge of the calorie content of food intake, i.e., knowing which foods are highest in protein content or the length of time required for various foods to digest, is by no means a "complete diet of healing" or sufficient qualifications for the nutritionist. Unless we recognize the tremendous importance of a thorough and "deep" cleansing of the human cesspool, we can very easily become deceived by Nature. This hitherto unexplained "ignorance" regarding the "fruit diet" has proven to be the "stumbling block" for all other nutritionists and "food research experts." Without a preliminary cleansing of the stomach and intestines of the mucus and decomposed protein foods stored in the tissues—eaten since early childhood—these poisons (i.e., cyanide of potassium) are dissolved too rapidly by the fresh fruits—and if permitted to enter the circulation in their concentrated form, cause severe sensations; yes, even death may result. And human's finest natural foods, i.e., grapes, apples, peaches, apricots, oranges, grapefruit, bananas, pineapples, figs, dates, and a host of others, are wrongly blamed! "Food experts" without exception give the advice: "Yes, you require more protein to overcome your weakness." This faulty advice is partly the "tragedy of nutrition."

The Great Event

During many personal tests involving this same problem, I tried vainly to overcome the "stumbling block" hundreds of times. After living for years on a "mucusless diet" combined with fasting, while traveling in Italy, I ate two pounds of the sweetest vine-ripened grapes and at the same time, I drank two quarts of freshly pressed grape juice. Almost immediately, I had the sensation that I was dying—extreme dizziness, heart palpitations, followed by severe pains in the region of the stomach and intestines! My vision became affected and I was forced to lie down. After about 10 to 15 minutes, the great event occurred. A mucus-foaming diarrhea together with copious vomiting and acid-smelling mucus—and this was soon followed by the greatest event of all! A feeling of great strength tempted me to perform the knee-bending and arm-stretching

26

exercises, which I did without tiring for 326 consecutive times! Prehistoric humans, living on unfired foods in their Garden of Eden, must have had this similar feeling. The tragedy of human existence, now easily recognizable, must be eliminated before humans can again ascend to this "paradisiacal" health! The Garden of Eden was a fruit orchard—and humans have been tricked through a wrong civilization, into unconscious suicide; reduced to slavery through producing wrong foods! This has now been going on through thousands of years, yet humans stubbornly refuse to acknowledge that their unnatural foods are the direct cause of all their sickness, untold suffering, and premature death!

"PEACE ON EARTH"—the end of all wars—happiness and righteousness—remain a foolish dream! During thousands of years, God, Heaven, Paradise—Sin, Devil, Hell—seldom found an interpretation that a clear, reasoning, mind would willingly accept. We are taught to believe that an all-forgiving Father will allow humans to enter Paradise in another world, unpunished for any of the violations of His laws in Nature. I have proven for the first time in modern history that a paradisiacal diet of fresh fruits is not only possible, but that it is an unconditional necessity for the rehabilitation of a degenerate humankind, such as we now find ourselves! It is the first step to real salvation and redemption from the many ailments and miseries of life. This, then, is the key to the "lost Paradise" where disease, worry, and sorrow—hate, fighting, and murder were unknown—a condition, at least, where there was no death from unnatural causes!

Nutritional Deficiencies

The adulterated, unnatural, false, man-made foods of present-day civilization are the underlying, physiological causes of all evils to which humans are prey—especially of all kinds of diseases. Health will not return, nor can it be regained, through drug remedies or the various treatments, since supreme, absolute, paradisiacal health is ruled by the laws of diet! All other methods must be classified as "aids" and come under the category of "assistance." Humans—like every plant and living organism—receive their growth from

27

childhood to maturity from their food, and their health or their disease is dependent upon the type of food they eat. The "Fall of Humankind" was therefore a "sin of diet." The paradisiacal story of eating the "apple" is misunderstood. The biblical use of the word "apple" was merely as a symbol of "food," for the apple in fact is the ideal food—king of all fruits, the real "bread" of heaven.

It required 4 to 5 years of continuous study, testing, and experimenting—oft times dangerous—for me to learn this truth! Nature wants to save you from whatever illness you are presently suffering. Regardless of how miserable, sick, feverish, weak, or desperate you may feel, you may depend upon it that Nature never loses interest in your welfare! Disease is merely an effort on the part of Nature to start performing the process of healing—to eliminate surplus waste and disease matters from your system. If you would but listen and heed Nature's still voice, i.e., "Remain quiet, rest, sleep, and *stop eating* so as to give me a chance to eliminate poisons and repair your bodily mechanism! Take time to be "sick" for a few days, and I will help you!" Thus, the instinctive voice of Nature speaks to all of her children, both animal and human! But Nature is helpless when you insist on obstructing her good intentions through drugs, "pain-killers," or increased eating.

If the waste-mucus and poisons in your already "overloaded" body are too great and of too long standing, then Nature cannot help—even fasting indefinitely is hopeless! You must eventually expire, just as do the wild animals that are beyond help and cannot recuperate through fasting alone. Nature's tendency of evolution is the final goal of "Quality" not "Quantity"—and the weak and degenerate are wiped out through nature's inflexible methods. This, of course, is true especially of those who stubbornly persist in violating all natural laws of living! While all natural healing methods and treatments are more or less cleansing, "healing" per se, they unintentionally or perhaps purposely seem to overlook the original source of the cause of the disease. The foods of today's "accepted diet" are presumably harmless and therefore permissible according to their reasoning, and so they fail to even suggest a discontinuance of their use!

28

The Value of the Fast

The animal kingdom exemplifies the wisdom of natural living through practical demonstrations. When an animal becomes sick or injured, it instinctively uses Nature's divine, curative law of fasting, contrary to accepted medical practice. Eating "nourishing foods" during the "critical" period is a fallacious practice, causing more harm than good! We soon recognize that humans are the sickest animals on earth through their incorrect belief in their "imaginative power" of a superior knowledge of food preparation!

Volumes have been written on the subject of fasting by self-styled "experts," yet there is no one who understands exactly what physiologically and pathologically takes place when the healing "holy" spirit, that is to say, the personal vital efficiency of the "unfed" body, definitely acts! Fasting is the most misunderstood and feared of all the curative agencies. Why is fasting so difficult, so weakening; yes, one might say, so dangerous; and why so doubtfully accepted? And my answer is this simple, mathematical, physiological formula, viz, "V" (vitality) equals "P" (power) minus "O" (obstruction). Absolute, vital efficiency is equal air-pressure minus obstruction (mucus). Physically seen, the human body is an "air-gas" engine, very similar to that of all other "air beings"—who exist a relatively long time by air only—generating absolute activity without solid or liquid food of any kind whatsoever during their entire existence! "Air pressure" or "air power" being the same at sea level everywhere on this earth, the vitality of all humans wherever they might be dispersed around the globe should be the same at sea level! The vitality of all humans should be the same throughout their entire lives, but unfortunately this is not so—and the only explainable cause can be through the difference of resistance, which undoubtedly results from the varying quantities of obstructions of "waste matters," i.e., "mucus" acquired through years of wrong diet: decayed, unused foodstuffs, proven and thoroughly explained in my book *Rational Fasting for Physical, Mental, and Spiritual Rejuvenation*.

We therefore find that the more clogged the system might be with "mucus," the less the vitality! When solid foods of all kinds are discontinued during a fast, the bloodstream, which by the way circulates throughout the entire system every thirty seconds (120 times every hour), starts dissolving the waste matter "mucus," which has been deposited in the tissues—especially in the stomach and intestinal tract but more particularly the specific organ where the symptoms of the respective ailment are located. Should the whole "constitutional encumbrance" cause the patient to be too heavily "overloaded" for their limited vitality, the overtaxed body is unable to handle the situation without causing the patient to become extremely tired, weak, and mentally troubled! Fearing death, the "sick human" understandingly lays all blame on the "lack of food!" It is at this point that a critical "stumbling block" arises for almost all fasters. No faster dies through lack of food—they actually suffocate in and from their own wastes! Awareness of this fact and proper preparation through living on a well-balanced, carefully selected diet will succeed in making the cleansing fast a pleasure rather than an unpleasant experience.

The length of the fast and even the "timing" between the shorter fasts—and instructions on the proper variations of the kinds of food to be eaten between fasts—should be individually applied in each case. This is especially true in cases of severe illness or long chronic conditions, where the patient's limited vitality is practically depleted and at an extreme low ebb. These precautionary methods must be carefully observed, since the quantity of "mucus" now being dissolved may prove to be greater than the patient's "vital efficiency." For this reason, the more slowly you proceed and the more time you have available, the less *vitality required* and the more certain the "cleansing" will be. So, may I repeat: the tempo, length of fast, and the choice of meals eaten between fasts should be carefully determined.

Eighty percent of the "chronic sick" whose condition has become serious would probably die from a *long* fast! For this reason, I consider the utmost caution necessary; in fact, I believe it would be a crime to recommend a long fast to any unfortunate whose sick organism is so greatly clogged with "waste" that vitality has practically reached a vanishing point! Just as an example: A long "transition diet" is necessary for the individuals who from early childhood were given drug remedies for their various ills suffered during a lifetime, whether through "innocence" or plain "ignorance." The harmful properties contained in these drugs are ever present, and take years for complete elimination!

A "special" selection of food is probably indicated, not for better nourishment, but for a "less aggressive" effect in dissolving the mucus and poisons, thereby avoiding a too rapid elimination of the waste obstructions which could result in becoming a dangerous situation.

Through this discovery of the tragedy of modern nutrition, all errors of science must be recognized and overcome, for humankind of today suffers more illness than they have during the past 20 centuries of Christianity! No other animal violates Nature's laws through gluttonous eating as does civilized, modern humans! In fact, humans have completely overlooked the foundational teachings of Christianity, the religion of love—through failure to recognize and abide by nature's fundamental teachings, i.e., the proper care of the human body! Our record of "self-destruction"—both through needless, cruel warfare and a "self-destruction," which inevitably results from the present-day diet of civilization— is almost overwhelming!

Christ said, "Truly I tell you, who is not regenerated by water and spirit (i.e., "spiro"-air) will not enter the kingdom of heaven." We still hopefully look forward to the "return of God's kingdom" by praying, or by the ethical, self-made morals or belief in miracles and transcendental existence! God's "heaven on earth" was once in the Paradise—the Garden of Eden,—which clearly means human's living, human's eating, human's happiness, human's absolute health has existed and can only exist among fruit-bearing vines and trees! The real physiological truism of the above statements mean the new, God-like people of the Paradise can only return through physiological purification—the salvation of healing from the sins of a "civilization diet."

31

Disease is internal uncleanliness, acquired over all of the ages through wrong foods! We find medical drugs have acquired the status of a "household necessity" today for the suppression of pain of the various symptoms. We cannot spare the necessary time to properly cleanse our ailing bodies through Natural methods! Drugs act instantaneously! Or perhaps they still "doubt"—despite the logical proofs presented! Humans do not lack strength—they lack Willpower! But eventually an accounting must be made! The more intelligent a human being becomes, the more careful they are about their diet. A "spiritual blindness" has driven present civilization to "fancy" foods, but time is running short and it is rapidly becoming alarmingly necessary that we must soon establish a diet regime according to our bodily requirements. We must close our ears and our minds to the false prophets posing as "experts," who ignorantly recommend "man-made foods" that are slowly but surely hastening our end. Civilization cannot exist much longer in our present manner, and we have already entered the age of dissolution of our present civilization!

Return to Paradise!

Original humans were placed by our Maker in a paradisiacal garden until a devastating sin, symbolized by the eating of the "apple," overtook them! God provided "invisible food" for humans; perfume from trees and flowers and other vegetation; pure, clear sparkling water, unpolluted and free from chemical additives and poisonous gases; magnetic impulses received through contact with the clean soil; electric vibrations communicated through the luxuriant growth of hair on the head as well as the body, for each single hair is an electric-receiving station. Direct, life-giving rays were received from the sun on the naked body. These "invisible foods" for the body and "spirit" are inexorably interconnected, and the "spirit" is of first importance; for this is the REAL human! Compare this with our present-day food, which is either damaged or whose food value is completely lost at the source of supply through processing—and even our organically grown foods do not escape the damage!

Our present-day source of essential "food supply" has become polluted, resulting in the many diseases and bodily ailments afflicting present-day humankind. But hopefully, we may still have time to readjust to Nature's guidelines and reinstitute the Garden of Eden! Humans may hopefully re-acquire the enduring vitality to live for hundreds of years at full vigor—just as they did when first put on earth and while living in Paradise, but they must inevitably return to a fruit diet. Does not the Bible tell us,". . . and the earth shall be inherited by the meek and humble." With human's change in food and natural living will come a spiritual regeneration. The cleansing must be two-fold, i.e., both spirit and body.

Only the inspired person can understand the fruitarian preference, which is the food of Paradise. We live in an age when humans are in open rebellion against Nature—which probably means that only a chosen few will listen and reap the benefits of Nature's teachings. Through the carnivore diet accepted by humans during the past centuries came the lowest physical form of living for humankind; actually killing and eating their co-creatures!

Nature's Warning Voice

Nature will not tolerate persistent, continuous abuse without exacting a penalty! The simple truth is oftentimes more difficult to believe than the wildest fiction. Plain facts appear incredible, yet statistics prove hundreds of millions of humans throughout the civilized world today are depleted in vitality and live only half-useful lives. Neither religion nor a university education can create vibrant health and radiant vitality. You can regain and retain health through a mucus-free diet (consisting of fruits and starchless vegetables), exercise, breathing, walks, and proper daily eliminations, fresh air, sunlight, and pure water! These are the curative agents. Allow Nature in her own way to repair and restore the ravages of disease, slowly but surely. You cannot expect worthwhile results if the cause is permitted to remain. The act of digestion begins as soon as food enters the mouth, but excessive quantities of foods such as meat, fats, and starchy foods make impossible the process of complete digestion. Instead of heeding Nature's warning voice to "desist," we

33

eagerly continue our wrong eating habits. Progress comes through recognition of sickness as a remedial measure. During 15 years of experimenting and tests carried out on my own body as well as hundreds of others, all of whom had previously received either medical or natural treatments, suffering from so-called "incurable conditions" (i.e., deafness, partial blindness, and paralysis), when using my methods of overcoming disease through corrective diet, all received complete results. "Disease is internal uncleanliness," and this message is deepened and glorified as the infallible truth through my conception of physiological religion!

When conditions for nutrition are ignored, the organs of life wither, waste, and weaken. Only through proper digestion can life be augmented through this physiological process. Changes inevitably must occur in the perishable substance—and putrefactive and fermentative changes are going on continuously. Decomposition of food in the stomach and small intestines is easily recognizable. Digestive juices, which the normal individual secretes every 24 hours, are estimated to weigh approximately 25 pounds, and these juices are poured back and forth during the digestive process. When these liquids are retained beyond a normal length of time, they cause inflammation—and bring about a pathological condition, a direct cause of nervousness. The intestinal canal and colon are used as a storage place, and the bloodstream absorbs poisons from this decomposing excess waste. We should free the bowels of waste gases and fecal matter as many times a day as we eat.

Fundamental Causes of Disease

Medical authorities inform us that we are rapidly becoming a "toothless" race through improper nutrition, with which I completely agree; and may I add that we are rapidly becoming an aggregation of "corpse colored" beings that we boastfully refer to as the "white race"! Western civilization can only receive a new lease on life through following the basic laws of Nature, i.e., the wise and proper use of fasting and a "mucusless-diet"! The *Mucusless Diet Healing System* requires considerably more detailed study than can be covered in this article. We have now learned that the fundamental cause of disease is the presence of foreign matter in the body—undigested, uneliminated, and putrefying food substance resulting from overeating, especially of mucus-forming foods. This disease-producing material is a partially digested, decaying, semi-liquid which enters and poisons the bloodstream through re-absorption and feeds these poisons to the various organs of the body. It is really proven that every person living on the accepted present-day "mixed diet" consisting of meat, starches, and liquids—or on a starchy vegetarian regimen—has a system more or less clogged up with mucus. It has long been recognized that meats and animal fats are not suitable for humankind. They cannot be fully digested, remaining in the tissues of the body as a sticky, gluey consistency, which eventually clogs the entire circulation. It is reasonable and self-evident, therefore, to assume that unless a change is made from their disease-producing diet—replacing mucus-forming foods with tree-ripened fruits and starchless vegetables—favorable results cannot be expected. The amount of mucus and toxic poisons stored up in the deepest tissues of the body is much greater than supposed. Care must therefore be taken not to allow the elimination to become too rapid while being dissolved through a mucusless diet. This is the probable explanation of why a radical "fruit cure" or a "long fast" without necessary knowledge of when and how to discontinue the fast often cause serious impairment of an already weakened vital energy.

Recapitulation:

The "tragedy of nutrition" remains a mystery to all those who refuse to believe that the nutritive and curative values of fresh fruits and starchless vegetables are far superior to all other foods. They not only furnish the blood with the best nutrient elements and dissolvent, but also starchless, green vegetables contain high mineral-salt contents and also enjoy valuable vitamins. We find the sick person almost forcibly fed on "mucus-forming" foods (i.e., eggs, milk, meats, and starchy "pap"). The formation of mucus continues, never ceasing until finally decay takes over and the bacilli make their appearance when death becomes inevitable. The "mystery" of the bacilli can be readily solved, thusly: The gradual clogging up of the blood vessels leads to decomposition of these mucus-forming products. Now, everyone surely knows that all meats, cheese; in fact, all organic matter will germinate in a favorable environment, putting forth bacilli during the process of decomposition. This condition of decay actually takes place in the living body and is referred to as pus abscesses, lupus, tuberculosis, syphilis, etc. The germs appear and are detectable only in the more advanced stage of disease. They are NOT the cause—but a product—of the disease, and disease-furthering because of the excretion of the bacilli and then toxins. I maintain that if humans lived in accordance with natural dietetic laws, on a mucusless diet, they would experience absolute health, beauty, and strength with no pain or grief—just as we are told in the Bible.

The seemingly healthy person must first pass through a condition of "cleansing" *sickness,* so to speak, or at least an intermediary stage of sickness, before attaining the higher level of health. *Properly,* humans in perfect health should exhale fragrance! The stench of odor, sweat, foul breath, and all body odors are merely indications of the rotting matter with which practically all bodies are weighted; handicapped almost from infancy to that final excess of corruption, which stills forever the human engine. *Red* is the visible color of life; *white,* pale, colorless, a token of disease. We have come to visualize old age as a state of decrepit old men and women. Ask any young person in their teens or even early twenties if they would like to become 80 or 90— and the answer is more than likely to be a horrified—NO! Becoming a centenarian is looked upon as being "unnatural." My *Mucusless Diet* holds forth a promise of longevity with every single day a thrill and joy of living that God intended for all of his children.

Why do we start growing old at 40? The answer must be— "through eating the refined foods of the conventional American diet"! Millions will needlessly die from various, unnecessary ailments, many before they attain the age of 75! And 80 percent of those who reach 65 will be invalids, suffering from catarrhal conditions, rheumatism, arthritis, Bright's disease, diabetes and many others— requiring hearing aids for deafness, and wearing glasses for failing vision, false teeth for loss of teeth; crutches, canes and wheel-chairs.

THE TRAGEDY OF NUTRITION—the cause of our failure to attain 65 with a healthy glow to our skin, vital energy, and ambition—and with never a thought of a complete cessation of all the worthwhile activities of life! Small wonder that hardening of the arteries starts at 50, when we deliberately dope our bodies with alcoholic drinks, nicotine and coal-tar poisons of cigarettes; caffeine from coffee and tea, meat, and mucus from starchy mucus-forming breads, cake, and cereals, all of which clog our bodies, eventually entering the bloodstream! Internally, we are all identical, with 30 feet of intestines. Study your own body—hunger for health knowledge; there are no secrets! Convince yourself of the absolute truthfulness of a mucusless diet! Our greatest desire in life is retaining "youth"—with its grace, beauty, vivacity, and charm! Through wrong eating, gluttony, and faulty elimination, we will be old at 40! This is truly

"THE TRAGEDY OF NUTRITION!"

- FINIS -

ABOUT PROF. SPIRA

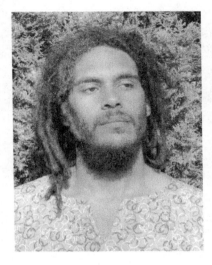

In 2002, Prof. Spira was a 280-pound former high school football player suffering from multiple ailments such as daily migraine headaches, allergies, regular bouts of bronchitis, sleep apnea, persistent heartburn, etc. After having lost his mother to a terrible string of chronic illnesses when he was in the 6th grade, he grew up assuming that he was genetically destined to be sick his whole life. While studying jazz trombone performance at the University of Cincinnati's College Conservatory of Music, he met a jazz drummer named Willie Smart (aka Brother Air) who told him about Arnold Ehret's *Mucusless Diet Healing System*. Within 6 months of reading the book, Spira lost 110 pounds and overcame all of his major ailments. He was able to throw away his CPAP unit (an oxygen mask that treats sleep apnea) and the medications he'd taken since childhood. Since his transformation, Spira has helped and inspired numerous people to use the mucusless diet to overcome their illnesses through his writings, music, and one-on-one consultations.

Spira is a professional jazz trombonist, educator, and author. He holds an MM in jazz trombone performance, an MA in African American and African Studies, and is a Ph.D. candidate in ethnomusicology at the Ohio State University. He is also the co-leader of an all-vegetarian and Ehretist jazz group entitled the Breathairean Ensemble, whose members are dedicated to inspiring their listeners to pursue what they call "physiological liberation." In 2013, Spira published his first book about the mucusless diet entitled *Spira Speaks: Dialogs and Essays on the Mucusless Diet Healing System*. He is the webmaster of www.mucusfreelife.com.

List of Other Publications

PROF. ARNOLD EHRET'S
MUCUSLESS DIET HEALING SYSTEM
ANNOTATED, REVISED, AND EDITED BY PROF. SPIRA

After almost 100 years, the *Mucusless Diet Healing System* has been revised and annotated for twenty-first-century audiences!

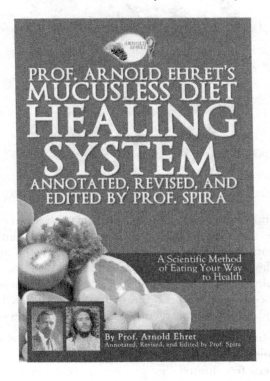

This is a must-read for all people interested in the Mucusless Diet!

Find it at www.mucusfreelife.com/revised-mucusless-diet

41

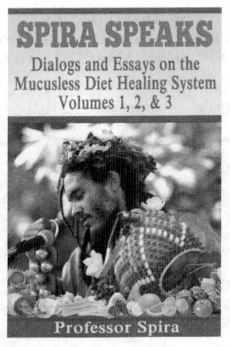

Join Prof. Spira for an unprecedented look into the healing power of a mucus-free lifestyle! After losing 110 pounds and overcoming numerous physical ailments, Spira learned that he had a gift for articulating the principles of the diet through writing and music. As he began to interact with health-seekers on the internet in 2005, he realized that written dialogs about the diet could benefit far more than just its intended readers. This book is a compilation of the best writings by Professor Spira on the subject.

What is the *Mucusless Diet Healing System*? How has it helped numerous people overcome illnesses thought to be permanent? What does it take to practice a mucus-free lifestyle in the twenty-first century? Why is the transition diet one of the most misunderstood aspects of the mucusless diet? Spira answers these questions and much more in his unprecedented new eBook that contains never-before released writings about the mucusless diet.

Visit www.mucusfreelife.com/spira-speaks

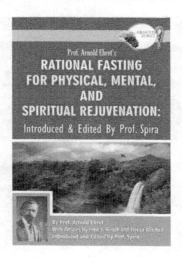

Discover one of Ehret's most vital and influential works, and companion the the Mucusless Diet Healing System. Introducing *Rational Fasting for Physical, Mental, and Spiritual Rejuvenation: Introduced and Edited by Prof. Spira*, now available from Breathair Publishing.

In this masterpiece, Ehret explains how to successfully, safely, and rationally conduct a fast in order to eliminate harmful waste from the body and promote internal healing. Also included are famous essays on Ehret's teachings by Fred Hirsch and long-time devotee Teresa Mitchell.

You will learn:

- The Common Fundamental Cause in the Nature of Diseases
- Complete Instructions for Fasting
- Building a Perfect Body through Fasting
- Important Rules for the Faster
- How Long to Fast
- Why to Fast
- When and How to Fast
- How Teresa Mitchell Transformed Her Life through Fasting
- And Much More!

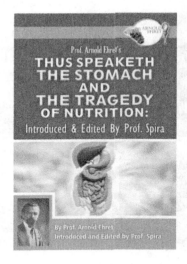
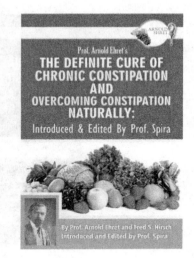

Thus Speaketh the Stomach and A Tragedy of Nutrition

If your intestines could talk, what would they say? What if you could understand health through the perspective of your stomach? In this unprecedented work, Arnold Ehret gives voice to the stomach and reveals the foundation of human illness.

The Definite Cure of Chronic Constipation and Overcoming Constipation Naturally: Introduction by Prof. Spira

In the Definite Cure of Chronic Constipation and Overcoming Constipation Naturally, Prof. Arnold Ehret and his number-one student Fred Hirsch explore generally constipated condition of the human organism.

COMING SOON!!!

The Art of Transition: Spira's *Mucusless Diet Healing System* Menu and Recipe Guide

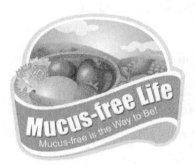

What does a mucusless diet practitioner actually eat? What kind of transitional mucus-forming foods are best? What are the most effective menu combinations to achieve long-lasting success with the mucusless diet? What are the best transitional cooked and raw menus? What foods and combinations should be avoided at all costs? How can you prepare satisfying mucusless and mucus-lean meals for your family?

These questions and much more will be addressed in Prof. Spira's long-awaited mucusless diet menu and recipe eBook! Stay tuned!

Introduction

Purpose

Popular Fruits, Vegetables, and Vegan Items Omitted from this Book

Organic vs. Non-organic

    Mucus-lean

    Raw vs. Cooked

Satisfying Nut and Dried Fruit Combinations

The Onion Sauté

Filling Steamed and Baked Vegetable Meals

Spira's Special "Meat-Away" Meal

Mucusless

Raw Combination Salads

Raw Dressings

Favorite Mono-fruit Meals

Favorite Dried Fruits

Favorite Fruit Combinations

Vegetable Juices

Fruit Smoothies and Sauces

Fresh Fruit Juices

Sample Combinations and Weekly Menus

Projected Release: Winter 2014

SPIRA'S MUCUSLESS DIET
COACHING & CONSULTATIONS

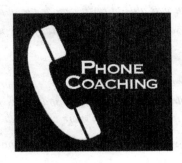

After receiving a consultation with Professor Spira, I was able to take my practice of the Mucusless Diet Healing System to a new level. Speaking face to face with an advanced practitioner was key and a true blessing on my journey. I'm looking forward to following up with another in the future!

-Brian Stern, Certified Bikram Yoga Instructor and Musician

You truly are amazing. You have done nothing but given all you can to help me and I truly appreciate this. Thank you for "feeding me."

-Samantha Claire, Pianist and Educator

"Spira has experienced cleansing on a higher level and passes those experiences to us. He teaches us by EXAMPLE and not only by WORDS, which is rare to find in the world we live in."

-Geargia Barretto, Brazilian Jazz Musician

"When I first contacted Professor Spira for help in practicing the Mucusless Diet, I had many addictions as well as obstructions in my system. I knew it would not be an easy road for me to get started, and I needed help. Professor Spira was able to give me the techniques I needed to start getting out uneliminated feces, black

sludge, worms, and mucoid plaquing from my colon and intestines. Within a year I was completely stabilized and elated to be a lifetime practitioner of the mucusless diet healing system. I felt that good! I also had gained the ability to take this system seriously. He then was able to further guide me in dealing with mental and emotional disturbances, social problems and holidays, as well as work and school issues.

His guidance was critical in helping me navigate a world of mucus, pus, and addictions. It has been almost three years now, and I have the vision and ability to practice steadfastly now, and I have much more work to do."

-Tony Bahlibi, Mucusless Diet Practitioner and Educator

Spira has practiced the mucusless diet and studied the natural hygienic/back-to-nature movements for the past 10 years. During that time, he has advised and helped many in the art of transitioning away from mucus-forming foods. For a limited time, talk with Prof. Spira about your individual needs, challenges, and questions. Skype, telephone, or in-person consultations available! For more information, visit:

www.mucusfreelife.com/diet-coaching

Visit the **MUCUSFREELIFE.COM** Amazon store for great deals on

Arnold Ehret's Classic Writings

WEB LINKS

Websites

mucusfreelife.com

breathairmusic.com

Facebook

Prof. Spira Fan Page: www.facebook.com/ProfessorSpira

Arnold Ehret Fan Page: www.facebook.com/arnoldehret.us

Arnold Ehret Support Group: www.facebook.com/groups/arnoldehret/

YouTube

Prof. Spira's Breathair-Vision: www.youtube.com/user/professorspira

Twitter

@profspira

@ArnoldEhret1

Visit our Bookstore to Find Books by Arnold Ehret!

www.mucusfreelife.com/storefront/

Spira is now available for mucusless diet consultations/coaching!

www.mucusfreelife.com/storefront/product/mucusless-diet-coaching/

Please Share Your Reviews!

Share your reviews and comments about this book and your experiences with the mucusless diet on Amazon and mucusfreelife.com. Prof. Spira would love to hear how the text has helped you.

PEACE, LOVE, AND BREATH!

CPSIA information can be obtained
at www.ICGtesting.com
Printed in the USA
LVOW03s0346270418
575101LV00023B/1055/P